I0425450

Lose Weight Keto

Easy guide to starting the Ketogenic Diet:
Using Guaranteed Strategies and
Methods to Help You Lose Weight,
Burn Fat, and Rapidly Improve
Your Mental Health

By Gabriel Walker

Table of Contents

Introduction

With the tremendous benefits that come with adopting a keto diet, many people are turning into it. But adopting a keto diet lifestyle only makes sense and becomes easy when you know what to do. Hence, it is not enough to decide to follow the keto diet; you need to be guided appropriately to make sure you are on the right part.

The desire to adopt a keto diet is not surprising as keto comes with tremendous health benefits. From losing weight to curing a range of disease like epilepsy and heart disease, the keto diet has proven very helpful. Overall, it helps maintain a healthy lifestyle free of excess weight and health challenges of excess weight. Over the years, many people have come up with different kind of meal plans to lose weight. Of all these plans, the keto diet has proven very effective.

This is why this manual is here as a guide. It will hold you by the hand in helping you start your journey into ketosis. We have meal plans that you can try as you go on. All in all, this manual will also shed light on what is ketosis and direct you on how to get there. Bear in mind, the ultimate goal of everyone adopting the keto diet lifestyle is to get to ketosis.

We urge you to remain faithful with the recommended ketogenic meal plans approved in this book. For it is when you are committed to the suggested meal plans that you can enter ketosis and reap the reward. All in all, get ready for a life changing experience that you will experience from adopting the keto lifestyle.

The keto diet involves adopting a meal low in carb, high in fat and with moderate protein. This could be pretty challenging for a couple of people. This is because there are challenges that will manifest as various signs when the body is transitioning into ketosis. Be rest assured this book is your ticket to ease the transition and reduce the effects.

Get ready for a complete overhaul in your health as I take you through this life-changing process.

Welcome

Chapter 1: Understanding Ketosis

Over the years, the spotlight has turned on the keto diet. This is not surprising as it is a meal plan that comes with abundant health benefits. The keto diet, a high fat and low carb meal plan, can turn your body into a fat burning machine. The surge in popularity of this meal plan can be attributed to celebrities and Hollywood stars that use it to stay in shape. The keto diet comes with many benefits from increased fat burning, to slowing down weight gain, to controlling blood sugar and reducing blood pressure.

Bear in mind that a keto diet is not a new found concept. It has been around as far back as 1920, almost a century ago when it was used to treat epilepsy. Then, researchers discovered that with elevated ketone levels in the blood, there were reduced epileptic seizures in sufferers (John M, 2013). With this, the keto diet was adapted as a treatment plan for kids and adults who do not respond to epileptic medications.

Ketogenic was coined form the 'ketones,' which led to keto, the shortened form. These are small fuel molecules that serve as a substitute for sugar in the body during a shortage of blood glucose. The production of ketones begins when humans feast on reduced levels of carb. Ketones also come from fat and serve as a powerhouse for the entire body, the brain especially. The brain which serves as the coordinating center of the whole body uses a lot of energy which comes either from the glucose or ketones.

Ketones in the body are produced in the liver from fats. These serve as a source of fuel for the entire body, the brain, especially.

The production of ketones in the body is called ketosis, a state of metabolism that should be desired by many people who wants to lose weight. The fastest way to get the body to ketosis is by fasting; however, fasting (staying away from food completely) could be pretty uncomfortable. With a keto diet, however, one can get to ketosis and reap the many health benefits of fasting even without fasting.

Switching to a keto diet means that the body is not powered by glucose, but fat. Unlike many other low carb diets, keto diets revolved around these macronutrients which are the source of 90% of the body calories. A drop in the level of body insulin spikes up the level of fat burned in your body. This is because fats are readily available; hence, they become the source of energy. With this, you will hardly go hungry since you get enough energy to stay focused all day

When the body is low in carb, the body transition to a metabolic state known as ketosis. This is when the level of ketones in the body rises, and the body breaks down glucose.

To shed weight, it is essential to burn fat. Besides that, getting the body to a state of ketosis does not come easy. Hence, you need to make it happen consciously. This is why your level of carb consumption in a day should drastically reduce. Some foods come with very high levels of carbohydrate like a banana (27grams of carb); hence take note of these foods and others in its category, it is also important to point out that one does not get to ketosis overnight. You will need a couple of days, days of dedication to the keto diet before getting to ketosis.

All in all, the keto diet is a low-carb diet which allows people to burn fat quickly since you concentrate more on eating fats, rather than carbohydrates. With the keto diet, your meal should contain a dietary plan of

- Fat in 60 to 70%

- Protein in 15 to 30% and

- Carbs about 5 to 10%

Types of Ketogenic Diet

Bear in mind that there are various types of the keto diet. However, they all revolve around reduced consumption of carbs and increased consumptions of fatty foods. A few of the types of keto diets are:

Standard keto Diet: this is the most common type of keto diet in which you eat a meager amount of carbs, (less than 50grams) per day. The ideal proportion is 75% fats, 20% protein, and 5% carbs.

Cyclical Keto Diet: If you want to commit to a cyclical keto diet, you will follow the standard keto diet meal indicated above 5 to 6 days a week. The carb intake during these 6 days is usually less than 50 grams. On the seventh day, you can eat as much as 150 grams of carbs – called the carb refeed day. The idea behind this is to cut back on the side effect that comes with restricting carb for a long time.

Targeted Keto Diet: While you also go with the standard keto diet, there is a slight difference. The difference is that 30 minutes before a high-intensity workout, you take extra carbs. The reason for this is apparent – for optimum performance

Dirty Keto Diet: With dirty keto, you will follow the recommended ratio of fats, carbs, and protein as suggested in the standard keto diet. The difference, however, is that you are at liberty to determine where your macros come from.

People Who Should Avoid the Keto Diet

Despite the effectiveness of a keto diet in bringing tremendous improvement to one's health, there are some group of people who should avoid the diet

People with Type 1 Diabetes: Type 1 diabetes patients are dependent on insulin. A keto diet could get their blood sugar level to dangerously low levels, which is terrible.

People with Eating Disorders: When you concentrate on a meal plan that eliminates a particular food group, there is a possibility of relapse in people with a history of eating disorder. Although Keto has proven pretty effective in helping to treat binge eating disorder, experts do not recommend this (Moira L, 2018). To treat binge eating disorder, you need a moderate, adequate, and regular intake of food without unnecessary ration.

People without Gallbladder: If your gallbladder has been removed, going on a high -ad diet will not help. This is because the gallbladder houses the bile, the body part that helps with digesting fat

People with Multiple Sclerosis: There are indications that a keto diet might not be safe in the long run for people battling with multiple sclerosis. There could also be side effects like constipation and fatigue.

All in all, bear in mind that a keto diet will not cure all disease. Also, going for the keto diet does not give the license to concentrate on all kinds of fats – there are unhealthy fats. Be sure to stay safe while on the diet

The next chapter will shed light on why you should consider the keto diet and the tremendous health benefits that come with this diet.

Chapter 2: Benefits of the Ketogenic Diet

Many people do attempt the keto diet for the sole purpose of losing weight. However, the keto diet comes with many health benefits. Keto diet gained wide acceptance and recognition because of its effectiveness in bringing about remarkable health changes.

By adopting the keto diet, some remarkable changes happen in the body that conditions it for tremendous health benefit.

A couple of the reasons you should try the keto diet are:

Weight loss

This is the number one reason why many people adopt the keto diet. At the onset of the diet, the body loses weight because of loss of water that comes from reduced carb intake. Hence, the body turns on fats stored in the liver since the consumption of carb has been limited.

Reduction in carb intake also reduces the level of body sugar. This translates to steady energy levels in the body. Besides, once people get used to the keto diet, they have a constant energy level such that they do not need to snack every couple of hours. Users are fuller with a lower level of hunger hence, reduced desire to eat.

Since your meal intake has changed, the body now burns fat for energy since glucose is scarce in the body.

This is how it happens:

On getting to ketosis, the levels of blood sugar and insulin drops. With this, the fat cells in the body let go of the water they have been holding on to. This is why a lot of people notice a significant weight loss on starting with the keto diet.

After this, the fat cells are in a better position to get into the bloodstream where they can find their way into the liver. In here, they get converted to ketones. This process goes on as long as you are on the keto diet.

Better Control of Your Appetite

This is one of the benefits of reduced carb intake. Your rate of hunger drastically reduces, and you do not suffer cravings like before.

Many people trying the keto diet discover that intermittent fasting becomes very easy. This is possible since hunger doesn't strike as it does before. Hence, you can go about your daily activities without rumbling from your stomach that you have got to eat

Improved mental Focus

Quite a lot of people have reported better memory and improved focus after getting on the keto diet.

When you concentrate on healthy fats, alongside omega-3 commonly found in seafood like tuna, salmon, and mackerel, you get to have a better mood with high learning capacity. This is not surprising as a fair percentage of the brain (15 to 30%) is made up of DHA, a fatty acid that gets increased due to the presence of omega-3 fatty acids.

Besides, getting into ketosis helps produce beta-hydroxybutyrate, a type of ketone. This is known to support and improve memory function.

Besides, one of the main issues with carbs as a source of energy is that it causes a rise and fall in the blood sugar levels. Due to the inconsistency of the source of energy, it becomes tasking for the brain to focus for long.

Getting into ketosis, however, makes the body turn on ketone for food. The source is consistent. Hence, you can focus for long.

Insulin Sensitivity

Excessively high levels of body insulin results in insulin resistance in the body. This can be addressed by using a keto diet. When you take meals high in carb, you are making the body's level of resistance to insulin to rise.

A keto diet, on the other hand, turns down the level of insulin in the body. This is understandable as you are now taking more of fat, a macronutrient that requires less insulin.

With a reduced level of insulin, your body can burn fat because excess insulin level works against the breakdown of fat. Hence, even a few hours drop in insulin level in the body encourages the breakdown of fat.

Control of High Blood Pressure

The number of people dealing with high blood pressure increases by the day. The problem is not really with increased blood pressure; the issue is that high blood pressure sets the stage for other horrible health condition like stroke, kidney failure, and heart disease.

There are, however, studies that buttress the fact that with a keto diet, you can get high blood pressure down, especially in people with type 2 diabetes or overweight people. (William S, 2015)

Cholesterol levels

With the keto diet, user can experience an improvement in the levels of cholesterol. What happens is that LDL levels decrease while HDL levels rise – which is expected and healthy

To know if you have a healthy cholesterol level, the ratio of total cholesterol to HDL matters. You can get this value by dividing the amount of your entire body cholesterol by your HDL level.

Your cholesterol level is healthy if you have a value of 3.5 and below. There is research that supports the fact that you can improve your cholesterol level with the keto diet.

Increased Energy level

The body cannot store much glycogen. As a result of this, you need to continually keep the level up to maintain a reasonable energy level.

In ketosis, however, this is not necessary as the body already has more than enough fat to work with. Hence, when you get to ketosis, hardly will the body run out of fuel. This translate to an optimum energy source

How beautiful it is if you do not have the urge to sink into your bed to relax after lunch!

This is the keto lifestyle!

Potential Health Risk of the Keto Diet

As impressive as the keto diet is, it doesn't come on a platter of gold. There are a few potential downsides that intending dieters need to know. The main one is that the diet is pretty challenging to stick with. According to a study in the Journal of Clinical Neurology, researchers sought for the rate of compliance among people on the keto diet and got 45%. According to Nisevich Bede

"The diet is pretty hard to follow because it's a complete shift from what you're used to,"

This can be attributed to the fact that your carb intake is significantly reduced. This makes you really, really hungry. Although the hunger subsides after a couple of weeks into the fast

Users should also bear in mind that there could be the possibility of flu-like symptoms. These manifest as fatigues, headaches, etc. This is commonly known as keto flu. Since you shed a lot of water weight on starting the keto diet, there is the possibility of dehydration. This could make keto flu worse. This is why staying hydrated is very important.

Other common health risks are a deficiency in some minerals and vitamins, kidney stones, reduced density bone density, etc. The reason for this is because there will be nutritional deficiency when you eliminate some classes of food like legumes, fruits, and whole grains. When you are short on fiber, for instance, there is a high chance you experience constipation.

To get around these risk associated with the keto diet, we recommend planning your need very well. This is important to ensure that you are having an adequate intake of essential nutrients. This might be difficult to expect if you are not working with a registered dietician with vast knowledge in keto.

Some Mistakes to Avoid While on the Keto Diet

A ketogenic diet is a complete change of lifestyle. As a result, it could be a struggle for a couple of people attempting the diet. This is because there is an internal change going on in the body, alongside a change in lifestyle and eating habits.

Many people tried the keto diet and loved the effects, while other people, on the other hand, did not see any reasonable change. Lack of result might be attributed to a simple mistake while on a diet.

You might make a mistake if you are not properly guided, but the fact that you are reading this manual will guide you against such errors. Following the keto lifestyle is hard; hence, you want to make sure you are armed with the right information to make sure everything goes as expected.

With this in mind, we bring forth common mistakes that people are prone to while on the diet.

Using keto as a "Quick Fix"

One thing many people who want to adopt the keto diet need to understand is that it is a lifestyle. Hence, it will not work if you're going to use keto as a quick fix for your weight or other health issues.

This is not to say that there will not be changes or effect at all, but the changes will not be long term. Besides, if you have any substantial change, you cannot expect to switch back to your formal eating habits and expect the changes to last. Hence, falling right back to your old eating habits will translate you right back to square one.

There are various types of the keto diet. As explained in the previous chapter, you can attempt the cyclical keto if the standard keto proves too hard. Bear in mind you are committing to a lifestyle change, and you have to be ready to stick to it long term.

That is how it works

Staying Away from Fats

Over the years, we have been made to believe that fat is the 'bad guy.' However, the irony of the matter is that keto diet makes you eat fat to lose fat, yes it is an irony, but it works.

Many people might marvel at the number of fats they have to eat when they calculate their macros. This is expected as a transition into ketosis is only possible with a massive amount of fats. Ideally, you should eat around 75% fat. This is a high amount, we admit, but it is ideal for getting rid of stubborn body fats lurking around your body.

You should not be afraid of eating such amounts of fat. In the long run, you will see tremendous health benefits hence be sure to flow along with the basics of the diet.

Concentrating on the Wrong fats

Alongside the last point, you have got to be sure that you are eating the right fat. That you have to eat a large portion of fat is not a license to pop in all kinds of fats. Without a doubt, there are good fats, and there are bad fats.

Bad fats prevalent in today's society are processed foods; processed vegetable oils, etc. hence, be careful of these and avoid cooking with these oils.

On the other hand, we recommend saturated fats, polyunsaturated fats, monounsaturated fats, and trans fat -natural ones. These are the types of fats that will aid your journey into ketosis.

With these types of fats, you will be sure to get the necessary amount of fat requirements while staying away from bad fats.

Eating Excessive protein

Okay, you are staying away from carbs, and you thought to compensate it with the intake of protein. Yes, that is fine, but the issue with this is that you will not get what you want. With excess protein, the body will have a negative reaction during fasting.

The body needs a certain amount of protein while adopting the keto diet lifestyle. Excess protein will be converted to fats, which is not needed. Bear in mind that part of the reason for keto diet is to get rid of fat hence adding another food that converts into an excess layer of fat is not worth it.

To avoid this, just concentrate on your macros. Be sure to eat based on your macros, and there will not be any class of food in excess.

Not taking Enough Water

Adopting the keto diet will make your body lose a lot of water. This explains why you have to make it a priority to stay hydrated. However, many people do not really focus on this.

Keto diet makes you lose not only fluids but electrolytes which you can easily replenish via the intake of water. Water deficiency in the body will make the body store a lot of fat, which is against what you want to achieve.

Besides, you need to be updated to ensure that your body organs are in top condition, well equipped to go about their normal activities.

Even if you do not like drinking water throughout the day, you have to. With the keto diet lifestyle, we recommend a gallon of water intake per day. This does not need to be overwhelming, as small sips can quickly add up to this with time.

Not Adding Variety to Your Meals

Without a doubt, a keto diet already places some level of restriction on the classes of food you can take many people, due to this, restrict themselves to a certain set of food every time. However, this does not mean you cannot experiment with varieties of recipes, as long as it is keto friendly.

That is part of the reason you have this keto diet manual, to expose you to as many keto recipes as possible. It is understandable to like a few sets of food. However, for optimum result, you should mix things up. There are keto recipes which you will get to experiment with later in this manual. This will not make the keto lifestyle journey boring in any way.

Be sure to include low carb veggies and fruits as well. This is because all the recipes will not have vegetables.

Be sure to experiment with varieties. It could be worse to concentrate on the same set of food every time. The disadvantage is glaring, with time, you will get fed up

Obsessing With the Scale

We understand that the ultimate goal of many on the keto diet is to lose weight. Bear in mind that you did not pack all the pounds of fat in a day; hence, they will not leave in a single day. Besides, the weight loss process is a journey which will take its time.

Checking the weight every now and then is a recipe for disaster. This might get you discouraged when things do not move as planned. Significant weight loss happens over a days and weeks, not hours.

However, be rest assured that if you follow everything as laid down, the meal classes in the right proportion, keeping hydrated and following your macro intake, your weights will reduce gradually.

Hence, the best idea is to check your weight once a week, And if you cannot keep your excitements down, check it twice a week. This will help you see the progress you are making with this new lifestyle of yours.

These keto mistakes can surely be avoided. To be forewarned is to be forearmed. Be sure to keep them in mind as you plan for the new lifestyle ahead of you

Chapter 3: What is Ketosis and How to get to Ketosis

Over the years, the basics of many fad diets out there teach us to restrict calories, have more workouts, and reduce fat intake for us to lose weight. However, many people have realized that the result of this is hardly effective.

Since the rate of obesity is rising geometrically, especially in developed counties, there has been research into healthy ways to lose weight. One of such is the keto diet. As it has been established in previous chapters, the keto diet not only produces weight loss but other tremendous health benefits for people who follow it.

The keto diet instructs users to eat meals high in healthy fats, moderate protein, and a limited amount of carbs per day. The aim of this is to get users to a metabolic state called ketosis. Entering into ketosis is the highlight of the keto diet. This is because users will not get the health benefits of the diet without getting into ketosis.

What is Ketosis?

Ketosis is a state you get to as a result of following the keto diet. In the body, you get into ketosis when the level of glucose from carbs drastically reduces. This forces the body to switch to another source of fuel – fat. While many people dread fat because it has been associated with excess weight and heart disease, it is a good source of energy in the absence of carbs.

When glucose is not available to fuel the body cells, the body looks for another source of fuel. This is when it burns fat for the production of ketones. As soon as the levels of ketones in the blood get to a certain point, the body gets to ketosis. This fosters a quick and consistent weight loss until you achieve healthy body weight.

In summary, here is ketosis and how to achieve that:

- A drastic reduction in the availability of glucose in the body, and all its sources like fruits, grains, starchy veggies, etc.

- The body seeks for an alternative means to keep up with its function - fat. This comes from food like avocado, salmon, coconut oil, etc.

- Since the primal source of fuel is not available, the body burns fat, which triggers the production of ketones in the blood.

- When your blood ketone levels get to a specific state, the body gets to a metabolic state called ketosis

It is the liver that breaks up fats into glycerol and fatty acid through a process known as beta-oxidation. In the body, we have three main ketone bodies produced in the liver, which are water soluble. They are acetone, acetoacetate, and beta-hydroxybutyrate.

Furthermore, the body breaks down these fatty acids in substance that powers the body called ketones that travels through the blood. The body breaks down fatty acid via a process called ketogenesis. This triggers the release of acetoacetate, a particular ketone that supplies energy.

With this, your body is powered by ketones moving around the body. This changes your metabolism such that you can burn fat quickly. With the ketogenic diet, you get to remain in this fat burning state. Since you achieve this via a low carb diet, you can no longer eat foods like bread, cereals, grains, and other processed foods. You now concentrate on foods like starchy vegetables, fish and butter.

Many people wonder how long it takes to get into ketosis. This depends on a couple of factors, but mainly on how limited your carb intake in, alongside some other variables that are not in your control like medical history, genetics, body composition, and energy needs. However, in a couple of weeks, your body should get to ketosis if you follow the keto diet strictly.

Some Signs You are in Ketosis

It is easy for some people to ease into ketosis because they can adjust to the lifestyle in a couple of weeks, a month tops. This happens with a few negative symptoms associated with the early stage of ketosis. It is common for your body to react when entering into ketosis. This is because your metabolism is changing.

Popularly known as keto flu, it could be a challenge for people starting out on the keto diet at first. This triggers some side effect that could stay for a week or two. The bright side, however, is that this goes away with time. As soon as your body starts getting used to being in ketosis, the symptoms decreases.

A few of the things you will likely experience as your body transition to ketosis are:

- Excessive tiredness

- Difficulty sleeping

- Extreme cravings for sugar and carbs

- Digestive issues such as constipation and bloating

- Being irritable

- Headaches and migraines

- Bad breath

This is what the initial phase of getting into ketosis will look like. On the bright side, you will likely notice some health improvement with time. Your appetite will reduce, and many of the positive benefits of the keto diet we discussed in the previous chapter. Those are indications you have positively transition to ketosis.

Experts on keto diets have declared that nutritional ketosis is measured by the levels of ketones in the blood, which is usually between 0.5 to 3.0 mM. Some people have agreed that 1.5 – 3 mmol/L is "optimal ketosis," which will trigger weight loss. People differ in regards to the exact amount of macronutrient they need to keep them in the range specified while giving them the ability to feel at their best.

You can also measure the levels of ketones in the breath, urine, or blood to determine if you are in ketosis. There are many ways to do this:

Blood ketone Meter: With the use of test strips, you can get an accurate measure of the BHB ketones in the blood. They are pretty reliable, and you can get them online to help know if your macronutrient consumption is in the correct ratio.

Urine Strip Tests: there are cheap urine strips which you can use to measure ketone levels is simple to use and cost-effective

Breathalyzer: You do not need a piece to measure ketones through your breath. The result might, however, not be as accurate as of the other two above.

Simple Tips to get into ketosis fast

We have established that when the body gets into ketosis, the body turns on fat as its source of fuel rather than glucose. The breakdown of fat in the body fills the blood with ketones. These ketones exit the body via the urine.

Achieving a state of ketosis requires some effort. This is why this section will shed light on simple, ways to get your body into ketosis fast.

Increase Workout

You can enter ketosis by increasing your physical activities. This is because the more energy you use for your daily activities, the more food you will need to replenish it. With exercise, the levels of glycogen in the body gets depleted, which gets renewed on eating carbs.

With the keto diet, however, you will not be replenishing the glycogen store since your intake of carb is reduced. Bear in mind that it could take a little while for the body to get used to fat for energy rather than glycogen. This could express itself in the form of fatigue as the body adjusts.

Drastically Cut Down the Intake of carbs

Since the body does not get enough supply of carbs, it is forced to act on fat, instead of sugar, as its primary source of fuel.

Hence, in trying to get to ketosis, we recommend limiting carb consumption to at most 20 grams per day. This will foster weight loss, help keep your blood sugar level in check while keeping your heart in good condition.

Short term fasting Period

One of the easiest ways to get to ketosis is via fasting. Many people find out that between meals, they could get to ketosis. Intermittent fasting as well, a short term fast interval, might also induce ketosis

There are cases a doctor might recommend a long period of fasting. It is advisable to be in touch with your dietician before deciding on any prolonged hour of fast.

Kids with epilepsy are at times made to fast for at least 24 hours before they commence the keto diet. This helps ease the transition into ketosis and the reduction of seizures.

Increase Consumption of Healthy Fats

You can improve your ketone levels when you eat a lot of healthy fats. Most, if not all, ketogenic diets have 80% of their calories from fat. The type of keto diet employed in treating epilepsy has up to 90% of fat.

Bear in mind; however, excess fat intake does not translate to higher ketone levels. You also, need to concentrate on high-quality fats only since the majority of your meal is made of fat. We recommend fats from sources like oil butter, avocado oil, butter, lard, and tallow, etc.

If your goal of following the keto diet is to lose weight, be sure to reduce your overall calorie consumption.

Maintain Optimum Protein level

You need a certain level of protein as well, although in minimal quantities. The keto diet used to treat epilepsy patients has a very limited amount of carbs and protein to boost ketone levels. We, however, do not advise cutting back on protein because it is not a healthy practice.

You need enough protein to equip your liver with enough amino acid, which helps in the process of gluconeogenesis, meaning "forming new glucose."

This is the process in which the liver provides glucose for the organs and body cells that cannot use ketones for fuel, for instance, the red blood cells and part of the brain and kidney. Also, you need optimum protein level to keep the muscle mass intact since there is a drastic reduction in carb intake.

Bear in mind that losing weight will result in the loss of fat, alongside muscle. When you take adequate protein with your keto diet, you get to preserve your muscle mass.

To know your protein need while on the keto diet, do multiply your healthy body weight (in pounds) by 0.55 to 0.77 (which in kilogram is 1.2 to 1.7Kg). Hence, if your ideal body weight, for instance, is 100 pounds, you should aim for a protein intake of 55 to 77 grams per day.

Consume More Good Salt

There is a couple of misconception about salt. This has made a lot of people struggle with the right amount of salt intake. This can be attributed to the excess carb ration which pumps up our insulin level. The kidney holds on to sodium because of excess insulin, which leads to a high Sodium and potassium ratio.

The keto diet, low in carb, helps reduce our levels of insulin. As a result of this, the body gets to pass out more of sodium as waste. Through this, we can get low Sodium to Potassium ratio. You can increase your intake of salt via any of the following:

- Use enough pink salt in your meals

- Consume more of organic broth

- Use sea vegetables like nori and help in your dish

- Take cucumber and celery – they are rich in natural sodium and low in carb

Use MCT Oil

One of the essential ingredients to get you into ketosis fast is high-quality medium chain triglyceride (MCT) oil. This is because it encourages the consumption of protein, which will keep you in ketosis.

If your diet is full of long chain fatty acids, 85% of the calories will be from fat. With MCT oil, you can get this level down to 65%. This is because it is easier for the body to digest MCT into ketones and used as energy.

It should be pointed out that MCT oil is not the same as coconut oil. While MCT oil comes from coconut oil, it contains some compounds that make it stand out. You can cook with MCT oil and even add it to drinks

Chapter 4: Food to Eat and Foods to Avoid

There are many people without a clear direction on what to eat and what to stay away from while having the keto diet. This part of the book will shed more light on this. Being on a diet could be pretty hard, especially when you have no clue what you should eat and stay away from. We will give you an in-depth breakdown of the foods that can help you get to ketosis fast

Fats and Oil

When trying the keto diet, the bulk of your food will be fats; hence, it makes sense to start with it. In making your choice, keep in mind what you like and do not like. You can tweak fats in various ways to spice up your meals like sauces, dressings, etc.

The body needs fat to thrive, the right kind of fats. In a keto diet, we encourage some specific types of fats. There are various types of fats in different foods, but you can easily stay away from unhealthy fats.

Saturated Fats: Examples are ghee, butter, lard, and coconut oil. They are recommended.

Monounsaturated Fats: Samples are avocado, olive, and macadamia nut oils. They are also good.

Polyunsaturated Fats: We advise against processed polyunsaturated fats like margarine. However, you can take naturally occurring polyunsaturated fats found in animal protein and fatty fish.

Trans fat: these are processed fats that have been altered chemically. We advise you to stay away from these completely. All forms of hydrogenated fats like margarine should be avoided.

Monounsaturated and saturated fats like avocado, nuts, egg, butter, and coconut oil are stable chemically and do not trigger inflammation in many people. They are good.

There should be a balance between your omega 6's and omega 3's. Hence, focus on foods like tuna, salmon, shellfish, and trout. You can take a small fish oil supplement if you do not like fish. We also recommend krill oil as a substitute for omega 3.

Be careful about the amount of sea-based foods and nuts you take since their levels of omega 6 could be quite high. Foods in such categories are walnuts, sunflower oil, corn oil, almonds, etc. To keep your omega 's at the normal range: concentrate on fatty and animal fish, reduce snacking, and be wise with dessert items.

With essential fatty acids, the body gets the needed boost for its vital functions. The problem, however, is that when on a diet, they could be out of balance. Some fat and oil fit for a keto diet is

- Olive Oil

- Egg Yolks

- Avocados

- Avocado Oil

- Mayonnaise

- Cocoa Butter

- Coconut Oil

- Macadamia/Brazil Nuts

- Coconut Butter

- Butter/Ghee

Proteins

We recommend choosing a protein food source that is pasture and grass-fed. This is essential to limit intake of bacteria and steroid hormone. Below is a list of proteins that are fit and perfect for a keto diet. However, you should eat a regulated amount of protein.

As regards poultry, we recommend choosing dark meat if possible, because it contains much fat content, compared to white meat. Red meat does not have too much restriction. Be careful with sausages and cured meats as they could come with added sugars and processed ingredients.

In eating meat, you have to be careful of your protein intake. Excess protein in your diet could reduce the production of ketones in the body and an alternate increase in glucose production. The aim is nutritional ketosis. Hence, you need to be smart with protein.

Some proteins fit for the keto diet are:

- **Fish:** We recommend everything caught in the wild such as cod, catfish, mackerel, salmon, trout, flounder, halibut, tuna, salmon, and mahi-mahi. Be sure to concentrate on fatty fish.

- **Poultry:** Pheasant, duck, chicken, and quail.

- **Beef:** Steak, roast, stew meat, ground beef.

- **Pork**: ham, ground pork, tenderloin, pork loin, etc. be careful of added sugar and concentrate on fattier cuts.

- **Shellfish**: lobsters, oysters, mussels, squid, and crabs.

- **Offal/organs:** tongue, liver, heart, and kidney. Offal is an excellent source of nutrients.

- **Whole Eggs:** We recommend going for the ones from the local market. It could be prepared in many ways: poached scrambled fried and deviled.

- **Bacon and Sausage:** be sure to stay away from sugar or any extra filer additions by checking out the labels

- **Nut butter:** We recommend natural, unsweetened nuts, the fattier version if possible. This is macadamia nut butter and almond butter. Be smart with legumes as they are high in Omega 6.

For protein, always keep in mind that moderation is essential.

Vegetables and Fruits

We have as well made a list of fruits and vegetables fit for consumption while having the keto diet. It is important to note that some fruits and vegetables contain carbs in large quantity. Hence, it is essential to reduce the intake of such.

Vegetables are essential while on the keto diet. However, be careful about veggies as some come with high sugar content. Hence, you have got to be smart with your choice.

For a ketogenic diet, we recommend vegetables high in nutrient and low in carbs; in other words, the dark and leafy vegetables. Classes of spinach and kale also fit into this category.

We also recommend cruciferous vegetables grown above the ground, which are green and leafy. We recommend going for the organic type, though, due to the reduced level of pesticides. For vegetables that grow below the ground, be smart in consuming those. However, an idea of their carb level will be helpful.

All in all, there is no hard and fast rule when it comes to taking vegetables on the keto diet. You have got to be careful and mindful of the carb content. In adding any vegetables to your meal, be sure to **limit** these types:

- **Higher Carb vegetables**: Onions, parsnip, mushroom, and squash are in this category.

- **Berries:** This is blackberries, blueberries, and raspberries.

- **Nightshades:** peppers, tomatoes, and eggplants

- **Citrus:** lime, lemon and orange juice in water

- Completely Stay away from bananas, starchy vegetables, and large fruits like potatoes.

- All in all, it is a general fact that fruits and vegetables that grow underground come with a higher amount of fat. Hence, take them in a controlled and limited amount.

Dairy Products

There are dairy products that are fit for consumption while on the keto diet as well. However, the same rule applies, be mindful of the carb content since the idea is to have a reduced intake of carb in general, irrespective of the source.

Diary is an excellent addition to meals while on the keto diet. However, your levels of dairy must be moderate as you want to consume more proteins, vegetables with fats and oil.

We advise going with raw and organic dairy foods if you can get them. Dairy that has been processed does come with a magnified amount of carbs, which is not the best idea. Besides, we advise full-fat products over low fat or fat-free since the fat content will be high.

For lactose intolerant people, we recommend great aged dairy products since they have reduced lactose. Some dairy products fit to eat while having the keto diet are:

- Heavy whipping cream and Greek yogurt

- Hard Cheese such as cheddar, feta, Swiss, etc

- Soft cheese like blue, brie, Colby, mozzarella and Monterey Jack, etc.

- Spreadable like cheese, sour cream, crème Fraiche, cottage cheese, cream cheese, etc.

- Mayo alternative and Mayonnaise that has dairy

Dairy can be an additional source of fat while on the keto diet. With meals like sauces, fatty side dishes such as creamed spinach, etc. However, bear in mind that these classes of food lack in protein. Always remember this when eating them along with a protein meal.

A couple of people could have reduced weight loss while taking excess cheese. Hence, if you notice your weight loss has slowed, we recommend checking how much dairy you consume.

Nuts and Seeds

You can also consume a number of nuts and seeds on a keto diet, But as with other classes of food, be sure to be careful of the carb content. We recommend roasting nuts to get rid of any anti-nutrients. Stay away from peanuts since they are legumes and not recommended on the keto diet food.

With raw nuts, you can add flavorings to your meal. You might choose to consume them as a tasty snack. This is, however, not recommended if you are after weight loss. Your insulin levels will generally rise and slow down the rate of fat burning in the long run

You can get good fats from nut but be sure to remember that they come with carbs that can add up pretty quick. Besides, some nut also comes with protein.

- **Nuts can also be high in Omega 6 fatty acids**; hence, be mindful of the amount you are taking in. In general, go for nuts low in carbs. The following can guide you when it comes to choosing nuts for eating while on the keto diet:

- **Fatty low carb nuts:** You can eat brazil nuts, pecans, Macadamia nuts to supplement fats

- **Fatty, moderate carb nuts**: almonds, walnuts, peanuts, hazelnuts, and pine nuts will help supplement for flavor

- **Higher Carb nuts**: Stay away from cashews and pistachios because of their excessive carb content. With two handfuls of cashew, you get the whole carb you should eat in a day

Rather than regular flours, you can go for nuts and seeds. They are standard on the keto diet and very common with keto diet desserts and baked recipes. Nuts are commonly used in almond flours while seeds are conventional on flaxseed meals.

In baking recipes, you can employ multiple flours to get a good texture. You can also combine and try various baking methods to get reduced carb counts in your recipes. It is also vital to bear in mind that we have multiple types of flours that act differently. For instance, the body quickly absorbs coconut flours, which require more liquid.

Water and beverages

We present some common forms of beverages that are allowed and recommended while on the keto diet. However, you should limit the consumption of restricted beverages.

Bear in mind that being on the keto diet drains water from the body. You lose a lot of water weight at first, which could cause dehydration. This is common when starting out the menu. However, you need to be extra prepared if you are prone to bladder pain or urinary tract infections.

Usually, it is best to drink eight glasses of water. This is useful while on the keto diet, but you need more. Bear in mind that a large percentage of the human body is made up of water; hence, hydration is critical to survival and optimum function of the body organs.

You might want to go for keto coffee in the morning to boost your energy levels. While this is good, moderation is key as well. Be sure to go easy on the caffeine as well as it could stall your weight loss process. If you must take caffeine, we recommend not taking more than 2 cups a day.

It is important to note that keto flu occurs as a result of dehydration and insufficient electrolytes in the body. This explains why drinking enough water is not negotiable as well as replenishing your electrolytes.

A list of the most popular beverages while on the keto diet are:

- **Water:** this is your ideal liquid to curb hydration. We recommend still or sparkling water

- **Broth**: combined with vitamins and nutrients, it is an excellent way to replace your energy as it helps kick start your energy.

- **Coffee:** helps with focus and mental clarity. It can also help improve the weight loss effect of the keto diet

- **Tea**: gives the same results as coffee. However, we recommend black or green tea if you do not enjoy a drink

- **Almond/Coconut milk**: we recommend the unsweetened version to replace your diary beverage

- **Diet Soda:** We advise limiting this as it can lead to sugar spike and cravings.

As evident, the keto diet is not as restrictive as you might be tempted to believe. There is much food you can choose, and your dish is only as limited as your creativity. All in all, in whatever you want to choose, be sure to be careful of the level of carb. To a large extent, it determines if you will get to ketosis. On the other hand, we also have a whole list of foods that you should stay away from if you are on the keto diet. The next section discusses this.

Foods to Avoid on a Keto Diet

We describe the classes of foods that should not be eaten or found in your recipes when going on the keto diet.

Starch and all its form

In abiding by a low carb diet, staying away from starch is critical. In our food today, the most significant source of carbohydrate is corn and wheat; hence, be on the watch out for them. However, in avoiding starch, you have got to be wary of all forms of flours (except nut flours) and grains. Starchy vegetables like beans and tubers are off the table as well.

Some forms of grains you should get off your food lists are:

- Corn

- Rice

- Sorghum

- Millet

- Rye

- Oats

- Quinoa

- Wild Rice

- Wheat

- Bran

- Bulgar

- Durum

- Wheat berries

- Amaranth

- Spelt

- White flour

- Triticale

- Arrowroot

- Semolina

- Flour

- Cornmeal

- Cottonseed

- Cassava

- Lentil

- Manioc

- Modified starch

If you have to bake, you can use low carb baking with ingredients like coconut flour, almond flour, etc.

All forms of Sugar

Even when not on the keto diet, sugar is not so healthy for the body. Besides, it wreaks untold havoc on the body that moderation is vital. Now when on a menu like a keto, it is important to limit sugar intake to very, very minute quantities.

Besides, you need to be smart about sugar as it comes in many names. Hardly will you see a product where the manufacturer will spell out sugar directly as part of the ingredients. It is masqueraded in various fancy names and comes in different forms as well. They give sugar many fancy names so that you will not suspect the amount of sugar that comes in a product. Hence, when buying your next packaged food, be on the watch out for the following:

- Brown sugar

- Barbados sugar

- Castor sugar

- Coconut palm sugar

- Date sugar

- Golden sugar

- Icing sugar

- Yellow sugar

- Raw sugar

- Grape sugar

- Brown rice syrup

- Carob syrup

- Corn syrup solids

- Sounds like syrup—

- Palm Sugar

- Golden syrup

- Diastatic malt

- HFCS

- Muscovado

- Panocha

- Corn syrup

- Caramel

- Scant

- Treacle

- Malt

- Florida Crystals

- Powdered sugar

- Invert sugar

- Corn Sugar

Be careful of sugars listed as their scientific names. Watch out for the following names, and it sounds like a chemical, scientific mumbo jumbo:

- Diatase

- Fructose

- Glucose

- Ethyl maltol

- Fructooligosaccharides

- Isoglucose

- Glucose solids

- Glucitol

- Lactose

- Galactose

- Maltose

- Levulose

- Dextrose

- Disaccharides

Do not be deceived, sugar is sugar, regardless of any fancy name that they give it.

Stay Away from bad fats

Fats are not created equal hence, on your next trip to the grocery store, be sure to review the set of ingredients on the packet. This simple act can help you stay away from artificial trans fats and processed vegetable oil.

As much as possible, stay away from trans fat that is produced artificially. You will likely see them as "partially hydrogenated" oil or vegetable in short. Also, all processed vegetables oil and margarine should be highly limited. The means of producing these oils are very unhealthy – commercially, they are dissolved in a solvent under high heat, deodorizers, and bleach. They come from a science experiment and not stable under heat. Stay away from them as much as possible. Be on the lookout for the following:

- Anything hydrogenated

- Anything partially hydrogenated

- interesterified oils

- Diglycerides

- Monoglycerides

- Margarine

- Processed vegetable oils

- Cottonseed

- Rice Bran

- Soybean

- Corn

- Canola

The sad part is that these classes of refined vegetable oils can be found in many products. Be sure to stay away from trans fat and check the ingredient list. Don't check the nutrition facts label. Some products might still have artificial trans fat in trace amounts which might not be reflected in nutrition fact labels. Because trace amount can quickly add up hence, double check a product.

Some foods like butter and meat also have trace amounts of naturally occurring trans fat, and this is not a cause for concern. It is the artificial one that is your enemy, and not the natural one.

Chapter 5: 10 Delicious Sample keto Recipes

1. *Coconut Keto Coffee*

Ingredients

- Ghee – 1 tablespoon
- Coconut oil – half tablespoon
- Black coffee – 1 cup

How to prepare

Put all the ingredients in a blender and blend thoroughly

Serve appropriately

Recipe Notes

Servings: 1

Macros (per serving):

Calories: 179 kcal

Fat: 21 g

Protein, Net carbs, and Dietary fiber: 0 g

2. *Keto Frittata*

List of Ingredients

- Bacon – 4 slices

- Eggs – 6 large ones

- Baby Spinach – 4 ounces

- Shredded cheddar cheese – 1 cup

- Sliced mushroom – 1 cup

- Butter – 2 tablespoons

- Pepper – 2 tablespoons

- Salt – half teaspoon

- Heavy cream – a quarter of a cup

How to prepare

Preheat your over to 1800 C

Over the high heat, place a cast iron, preferably frying pan

Add your diced bacon and sauté into the frying pan.

Leave for about four minutes and add butter.

Get your sliced mushroom ready and pour in the pan

Sauté the entire mixture for about three minutes

Into the cooking mixture, add spinach and cook for two more minutes till it is wilted.

Remove from the heat and add some cheddar cheese into the pan

Get a mixing bowl, in it put cream, eggs, pepper, and salt

Whisk the entire mixture thoroughly till it is combines

Pour all the mixture into the pan and place in the over

Bake for 20 minutes

After this, it is ready for serving

Recipe Notes

Servings: 4

Macros (per serving):

Fat: 36 g

Protein: 21 g

Calories: 426 kcal

Total carbs: 3 g

Dietary fiber: Nil

3. *Lemon Black Pepper Tuna Salad*

List of Ingredients

- Dice one-third of a whole cucumber into small pieces
- Dice half of a small avocado into small pieces
- Lemon juice: 1 teaspoon
- Tune: 1 can
- Use salt and black pepper to taste
- Mustard: 1 tablespoon
- Mayonnaise: 1 tablespoon
- Salad green

How to prepare

With your cucumber already diced, mix it with lemon juice and avocado

Flake the tuna and mix with mayonnaise and mustard

Add the two mixtures together – tuna with cucumber and avocado

If you want, you can add salt to taste.

Serve and enjoy

Recipe Notes

Servings: 1

Macros (per serving):

Fat: 40 g

Protein: 45 g

Calories: 480 kcal

Total carbs: 11 g

Net carbs: 3 g

Dietary fiber: 8 g

4. *White Lasagna Stuffed Peppers*

List of ingredient

- Sweet pepper – 2 large, seeded and halved

- Garlic salt - 1 tablespoon

- Ground turkey – 12 ounces

- Mozzarella – 1 cup

- Ricotta Cheese – 1 cup

- Cherry tomato – 8 (optional though)

How to prepare

Raise your over to temperature as high as 205-degrees Centigrade

Put the halved sweet pepper into the baking dish and spread one quarter garlic salt in it

Unto the pepper, spread out the turkey. Sprinkle another quarter teaspoon of garlic salt.

Place the mixture in the oven and bake for about 30 minutes

Into the pepper, sprinkle the ricotta cheese and the mozzarella and the remaining garlic salt.

If you are using the tomato, slice it into the mixture

Bake for half an hour till the meat is well cooked, the pepper softens out, and the cheese becomes golden.

Serve into four plates and enjoy

Recipe Notes

Servings: 4

Macros (per serving):

Fat: 14 g

Calories: 281 kcal

Protein: 32 g

Net carbs: 6.5 g

Total carbs: 7 g

Dietary fiber: 0.5 g

5. *Shrimp and Zoodles*

List of Ingredients

- Butter – 1 tablespoon
- Shrimp – 1 pound
- Butter – 1 tablespoon
- Zucchini – 3 medium size
- Chopped garlic – 5 cloves
- Olive oil – 1 tablespoon
- Paprika - 1 teaspoon
- Lemon juice – 3 tablespoons
- Chopped parsley – a quarter cup
- Red Chili flakes – 1 pinch
- Pepper - ¼ tablespoon
- Salt - ½ teaspoon
- Use feta or parmesan for garnishing

How to prepare

You will need a zoodle device to make your zucchini. Spread it out on the double paper towels.

Spread a teaspoon of salt and roll up the towel.

Leave for a couple of minutes

Inside the pepper, add your shrimp, salt, paprika, and chili flakes

Get a large skillet, place over low heat

Add a tablespoon of butter and allow to melt.

Add a tablespoon of olive oil to the mixture

Add the shrimp and leave for about 3 minutes to cook and turn

Leave an extra 2 minute for the other side to cook

Remove from the skillet and put aside

Add garlic, red pepper, into the skillet and allow to cook for about 120 seconds.

Into the pan, add lemon juice and scrape it off the pan

Add the zoodles and sauté for an average of 4 minute

Into the skillet, add shrimp and some parsley

Stir while it is being cooked.

Serve into four plates

Recipe Notes

Servings: 4

Macros (per serving):

Calories: 210 kcal

Fat: 8 g

Protein: 25 g

Total carbs: 8 g

Net carbs: 6 g

Dietary fiber: 2 g

6. *Keto Homemade ham*

List of Ingredients

- Smoked boneless gammon – 2 pounds
- Chopped onions - 1 piece
- Chopped celery stalk – 1
- Garlic cloves – 1, bashed
- Black peppercorns – 2 teaspoons
- Whole cloves – 1 teaspoon
- Whole cinnamon stick – half
- Whole nutmeg – a quarter
- Salt – a quarter of a cup

How to prepare

Get a large pot, out the entire ingredients and add cold water

Boil the water and skim off the top foam with a spoon

Reduce the heat to the simmer, leave the pot cover ajar to facilitate slow evaporation

Simmer for 90 minutes

Leave for about an hour to allow the ham cool

Separate the liquid and place in a refrigerator.

It can be preserved for up to 7 days

Recipe Notes

Servings: 8

Macros (per serving):

Calories: 112 kcal

Protein: 20 g

Fat: 4 g

Net carbs and Dietary fiber: 0 g

7. *Fresh Bell Pepper Basil Pizza*

List of Ingredients for the Pizza base

- Mozzarella Cheese – 6 ounces

- Almond flour – half cup

- Psyllium husk powder – 2 tablespoon

- Egg – A large one

- Italian seasoning – 1 teaspoon

- Parmesan Cheese – 2 tablespoons

- Salt – half teaspoon

- Pepper – half teaspoon

List of Ingredients for the toppings

- Shredded cheddar cheeses – 4 ounces

- Tomato – a piece

- Marinara sauce – a quarter of a cup

- Bell pepper – two third

- Basil – 3 tablespoons

How to prepare

Preheat your oven to a temperature of 204 degrees Centigrade

Put the Mozzarella cheese in your microwave till it is melted

Put all the pizza base ingredients in the cheese and mix thoroughly

With a rolling pin, flatten the dough into a circle

Put the entire mixture in the oven for 10 minutes,

Get it out of the oven and spread the topping ingredient on top

Put it back in the oven and allow it to bake for an extra 10 minute

Recipe Notes

Servings: 4 (half pizza is 1 serving 2 pizzas of 4 servings.)

Macros (per serving):

Calories: 411 kcal

Fat: 31.3 g

Protein: 22.3 g

Net carbs: 6.5 g

8. Brownie Batter Mug Cake

List of Ingredients

- Almond flour – 1 tablespoon

- Flaxseed meal – 1 tablespoon

- Butter – 2 tablespoon

- A large egg

- Baking powder – half teaspoon

- Cocoa powder – 1 tablespoon

- Nut Zez Brownie Batter Almond Butter – one and a half tablespoon

How to prepare

Put the entire ingredient in a mug and mix

Microwave for about a minute

Leave it to cool and pour the content in a plate, leaving the mug upside down

To make the brownie flow out, tap the mug and enjoy

Recipe Notes

Servings: 2

Macros (per serving):

Calories: 242 kcal

Net carbs: 2.6 g

Fat: 23.3 g

Protein: 7.8 g

9. *Low Carb Cheesecake Brownies*

List of Ingredients for the brownie

- Salt – half teaspoon
- Almond flour – three quarter cup
- Erythritol – two-third of a cup
- Cocoa powder - two-third of a cup
- 2 large eggs

List of ingredients for the Cheesecake

- A large egg
- Vanilla extract – 1 teaspoon
- Erythritol – One-quarter of a cup
- Cream cheese – 8 ounces

How to prepare

Preheat the oven to 175-degree centigrade

With a parchment, line the bottom of an 8 by 8 pan

Spray cooking spray on the pan

Cream the sweetener and cream cheese together till it is smooth

Add the vanilla and egg and mix thoroughly till you achieve a cream and soft feeling

Melt the butter, add sweetener, salt, and cocoa.

Stir vigorously till the sweetener dissolves

As you stair, add the egg to the mixture one at a time

Add the almond flour slowly as you mix till it forms a good dough

Add two third of the brownie batter into your prepared pan

Dollop your cheese batter into the brownie

Pour the rest of the brownie batter.

Bake for like 23 minutes and keep an eye on it

Allow to cook and cut

Refrigerate it for about 10 minutes

It can be left in a refrigerator for 3 days

Recipe Notes

Servings: 16

Macros (per serving):

Calories: 155 kcal

Fat: 15 g

Protein: 4 g

Net carbs: 1.5 g

10.Loaded Cauliflower Mashed Potatoes

List of Ingredients

- Cauliflower – 1 head

- Garlic – 1 clove

- Butter – 3 tablespoon

- Salt – half teaspoon

- Pepper – one eight teaspoon

- Green onions

- Bacon – 4 slices

- Sour cream – 1 tablespoon

How to prepare

Heat a pot of water to boiling point and put the cauliflower in.

Reduce the heat and simmer for an average of 10 minute

Drain the water from the cauliflower

Get a food processor, add the garlic, pepper, salt, cauliflower, and sour cream

Process the entire mixture for about two minutes

Spread some cheese, green onions and crumbles on the top

It is best served warm

Recipe Notes

Servings: 4

Macros (per serving):

Fat: 22 g

Calories: 257 kcal

Protein: 7 g

Net carbs: 5 g

Chapter 6: How to Maintain the ketogenic Lifestyle

By now, you have all the tips needed for getting your body into ketosis. Bear in mind, and it is not enough to get to ketosis but to remain in ketosis as well. Hence, it is essential to arm yourself with crucial tips to help you maintain ketosis.

We discuss some of the essential tips below:

Concentrate only on keto Friendly Foods

The idea behind the keto diet is a meal very low in carb. However, the amount of low carb for the various individual is a factor of the daily carb limit. Hence, it is best to keep the net carbs below 25gram and total carb below 35 grams. This will enable you to reap the benefits of the keto diet.

Since your carb intake is limited, you have to be smart about food choices. Hence, you might have to ditch some of your favorite foods you have been used to over time. We do not even recommend all healthy fruits and vegetables. This is not to discourage you in any way, and there are other delicious recipes you will find interesting.

The previous chapters have done justice on the food that is recommended and not advised on the keto diet.

Track Your Macros

Many people hardly pay attention to the number of calories they eat. Besides, estimated calorie intake and actual calorie we eat is usually so different that we might be tempted to feel we are eating way less calorie.

We advise using a calorie tracking app and a scale to keep tabs on what you are eating. This method will help you know if you are consuming the right food amount as well as direct you on how to go about your weight loss.

You can get accurate info about the type of calorie you are taking by using a food scale. Many people base their calorie intake on guesswork, which can sometimes make you eat extensively. In buying a range, be sure to look for the following features

Presence of a conversion button: Most websites and calorie tracking apps use varieties of units. With a conversion button on your scale, you should be able to measure your food quickly. Most especially, we recommend going for a gram to an ounce or an ounce to a gram.

Tare Function: You should be able to have bowls, plates, and other utensils on your scale. This makes it easier to weigh things. There should be a tare function on it so you can place items on it

Removable Plate: There should be a removable plate to bring about easy cleaning. This is due to the possibility of having messy foods on your scale.

Tracking your food consumption the right way will help you focus on getting the result you want, keeping you in ketosis

Be careful of Your Environment

The type of food the world presents to us is way different from what our forefathers grew into. We are met with all kinds of foods that make it easier for the disease to attack and for people to pack excess weight. This was not what our forefathers had, which made it easier for them to have a long life and a lean body.

Processed foods are abundant in every corner, we watch it in commercials, and the smell attracts us. This triggers our brain to go for this tantalizing aroma, which comes so quickly. To make things worse, we eat way more than we need. This triggers weight gain. As a result of this, it is essential to do all in your capacity to make your environment keto friendly.

Some of the things we recommend are:

Keep only keto Friendly Food around: Hunger makes it so easy to cheat and feast on anything available. Hunger has a strong drive which acts irrationally and does not care about your weight loss goals. As a result of this, we advise you always to plan and make your home keto friendly. Let all carb-rich food be out of reach, and the healthy keto friendly food be within reach. Besides, keto food should want to go for should not require much preparation.

Always Plan Your meals Early: A plan makes it easy to stay on track and avoid temptation. There are keto friendly snacks and pre-made meals you can go for. All in all, your meal plan should give you the right amount of carb, fats, and protein in the recommended proportion

Avoid Easy foods that Might make You Binge: A convenient and tasty food is more natural to eat since it doesn't require much effort for preparation. Some people can go for an excess amount of a particular food, even keto food. As a result of this, we recommend not making an excessive amount of a food item at once. Hence, if it will be hard for you to control the urge to binge eat a particular food, restrict the amount you make such that making another will discourage

Concentrate only on Foods you can measure and track: Do not be tempted to include other instruments you will not be able to measure. It can get you off your macronutrient goals. A little extra oil and cheese here and there could shoot up your calorie to the point where it gets easy to gain weight.

Avoid Changing Your Plan Quickly

Your body will lose a ridiculous amount of water when you start keto, which manifests as weight loss. This will cause a change in the amount of calorie you need, and with time, there will be variation in the number of calories you need. With this, you will lose weight but not at a fixed pattern.

The implication of this is that some weeks will feel as if you are not losing weight. You might be discouraged by what the scale tells you. It is, however, important to stick with the plan as this helps long term weight loss.

You should aim for an average weight loss of 1 to 2 pounds per week. However, if you discover that you are not making encouraging progress, we recommend adjusting your lifestyle and diet choice. Take note of the following strategies

- Know your macro requirement and be sure it is deficient in calories. If you are after weight loss, make sure the deficit is high

- Make it a monthly strategy to calculate your macro needs monthly. Make this the plan you will stick with.

- Take breaks once a while from being in a calorie deficit, maybe once a week

- Track the food you eat and never cheat

- Attempt intermittent fasting

If the above strategy did not work, there might be a food allergy holding you back. Besides, it could also be that you are getting excess calorie from a hidden source.

Be Set for keto Flu and other keto Concerns

You have been so used to consuming carbs without restriction. Switching to a low carb food all of a sudden will be met with lots of revolt from your body. Many people will experience excess loss of minerals like sodium and water at first. Here are some of the keto flu you should prepare for dizziness, insomnia, confusion, stomachache, brain fog, irritability, nausea, and muscle soreness.

The best part is that by taking a lot of water, you will get rid of these symptoms. Hence, to be in ketosis for long, you have got to make it a habit to take lots of water

Use a Smart Meal plan

Following a meal plan is the best way to get and keep you in ketosis. This will reduce the overwhelming feeling from having to process all the info in this book. Here is a sample meal plan for three days, for instance:

Day 1
- Breakfast: A serving of Bacon Crusted Frittata Muffins
- Lunch: A serving of Spinach Watercress Keto Salad
- Dinner: A serving of Salmon Patties with Herbs

Day 2
- Breakfast: A serving of Bacon Crusted Frittata Muffins
- Lunch: A serving of Bacon Cheeseburger Salad
- Dinner: A serving of Bacon Cheeseburger Casserole

Day 3

- Breakfast: A serving of Hunger Buster Low Carb Bacon Frittatas

- Lunch: A serving of Spinach Watercress Keto Salad

- Dinner: A serving of Bacon Cheeseburger Casserole

Day 4

- Breakfast: 1 serving of Bacon Crusted Frittata Muffins

- Lunch: 1 serving of Bacon Cheeseburger Salad

- Dinner: 1 serving of Salmon Patties with Herbs

Day 5

- Lunch: 1 serving of Spinach Watercress Keto Salad

- Dinner: 1 serving of Bacon Cheeseburger Casserole

- Breakfast: 2 servings of Hunger Buster Low Carb Bacon Frittatas

Conclusion

The keto diet comes with many benefits. However, what turns many people away is that they will be limited in terms of meal intake. We have provided various forms of keto recipes in this manual. Hence, you can get creative and play around with it.

Besides, the keto lifestyle does not have to be a burden or a restriction. The aim of going into keto diet for many people is to lose weight and enjoy the many health benefits that come along with it. Hence, be sure to follow all you have learned in this book and be creative about how you eat. Diet plan gets boring, and many people find it difficult to stick with it when are restricted to tasteless meals.

Be sure to get your house in order in preparation for the keto lifestyle journey. Get rid of every food that is not keto friendly. If possible, ask your spouse or any of your housemates to join you in the diet. It gets easier if you are not alone. Besides, the absence of keto friendly food also removed the temptation of going above your daily carb limit.

While keto comes with a whole lot of health benefits, users need to be aware of the potential danger. We have listed some class of people not fit for the diet. Besides, if you are on any medication, be sure to talk to your doctor before starting the keto diet. In addition to that, be prepared mentally for the side effects known as keto flu. The good news, however, is that you can lessen the side effect of transition into keto by drinking a lot of water, this is not negotiable.

While the majority of food classes you will concentrate on is fats, be aware that there are good fats and bad fats. Hence, be sure to follow all the recommended ideas in this manual. We have listed bad fats you should stay away from. Keep them in mind, so they do not sabotage your effort to get into ketosis.

On a final note, be aware that you will not likely have the same result with other people, even your spouse if you follow the keto diet together. Keep this in mind, and do not be discouraged. The reason for this is due to the many variables present. Your body, your activity level, and your ages differ. The way you workout and the kind of lifestyle you lead all add to the variables. Be sure to stick to the plan and be faithful with it. When you get to ketosis, you will experience the tremendous health benefits of the keto diet.

References

Calihan J, (2018). Ingredients to avoid on a low-carb or keto diet. Retrieved from https://www.dietdoctor.com/low-carb/ingredients-to-avoid

Eenfeldt, A., (2019). A ketogenic diet for beginners. Retrieved from https://www.dietdoctor.com/low-carb/keto

Freeman J, (2013). Epilepsy's Big Fat Answer. Retrieved from https://www.ncbi.nlm.nih.gov/pmc/articles/PMC3662214/

Fletcher J, (2019). How to get into ketosis fast. Retrieved from https://www.medicalnewstoday.com/articles/324599.php

Hendon L. (2015). Lemon Black Pepper Tuna Salad Recipe [Keto, Paleo, AIP], Retrieved from https://paleoflourish.com/lemon-black-pepper-tuna-salad-keto-paleo-aip/

Joy Filled (No Date). WHITE LASAGNA STUFFED PEPPERS – LOW CARB KETO THM S. Retrieved from https://joyfilledeats.com/white-lasagna-stuffed-peppers/#wprm-recipe-container-13469

Laughing Spatula. (No Date). ZUCCHINI NOODLES WITH SHRIMP. Retrieved from https://laughingspatula.com/zucchini-noodles-with-shrimp/

Lawler M, (2018). Keto and Binge Eating Disorder 101. Retrieved from https://www.everydayhealth.com/ketogenic-diet/keto-binge-eating-disorder/

Levy J, (2018). What Is Ketosis? Hint: It Can Help You Burn Fat & Suppress Your Appetite. Retrieved from https://draxe.com/what-is-ketosis/

Migala J, (2019). A Detailed Guide to the Potential Health Benefits and Risks of the Keto Diet. Retrieved from https://www.everydayhealth.com/diet-nutrition/ketogenic-diet/what-are-benefits-risks-keto-diet/

Moodie A., (no date) Keto Diet for Beginners – Your Complete Guide. Retrieved from https://blog.bulletproof.com/keto-diet-beginners-guide/

Ruled.me, (no date). The Ketogenic Diet - A Keto Guide for Beginners. Retrieved from https://www.ruled.me/guide-keto-diet/

Ruled me. (no date). Ketogenic Diet Food List: Everything You Need to Know. Retrieved from https://www.ruled.me/ketogenic-diet-food-list/

Thrive Strive. (no date)., 7 Benefits of a Keto Diet That You'll Want in Your Life. Retrieved from https://thrivestrive.com/keto-benefits/

Spritzler F. (no date). The complete guide to ketosis. Retrieved from https://www.dietdoctor.com/low-carb/ketosis

William S. (2005). A low-carbohydrate, ketogenic diet to treat type 2 diabetes. Retrieved from https://www.ncbi.nlm.nih.gov/pmc/articles/PMC1325029/